# Paleo Diet Simple Guide for Beginners

## Paleo Diet for Special Populations

By

Nairne Oisean

# Table of Contents

# CHAPTER 1

# Introduction

## 1.1 What is the Paleo Diet?

The Paleo Diet, short for the Paleolithic Diet, is a dietary approach that seeks to mimic the eating patterns of our distant ancestors, specifically those who lived during the Paleolithic era, which began approximately 2.5 million years ago and ended around 10,000 years ago with the advent of agriculture. The fundamental idea behind the Paleo Diet is to consume foods that our hunter-gatherer ancestors would have had access to, and to avoid or minimize the intake of foods introduced with the advent of agriculture, industrialization, and modern food processing.

The primary focus of the Paleo Diet is on whole, unprocessed foods, with an emphasis on animal proteins, fruits, vegetables, nuts, and seeds. It excludes grains, legumes, dairy products, processed foods, and added sugars. The rationale behind this diet is that the human body is genetically adapted to the dietary patterns of our ancient ancestors, and by adhering to these dietary principles, individuals can promote better health, manage weight, and reduce the risk of certain chronic diseases.

## 1.2 Historical Background

The origins of the Paleo Diet can be traced back to the 1970s when it was first popularized by gastroenterologist Walter L. Voegtlin in his book "The Stone Age Diet." However, it gained broader recognition in the early 21st century with the publication of books such as "The Paleo Diet" by Dr. Loren Cordain and "The Primal Blueprint" by Mark Sisson.

The historical background of the Paleo Diet stems from anthropological and archeological research that examined the dietary habits of prehistoric humans. By studying ancient human remains, researchers have gained insights into the types of foods that early humans consumed. These studies suggest that the Paleolithic diet primarily consisted of lean meats, fish, fruits, vegetables, nuts, and seeds. Grains, legumes, and dairy were notably absent from their diet, as they were not yet cultivated or domesticated.

## 1.3 Principles and Philosophy

The Paleo Diet is built upon several core principles and a distinct dietary philosophy:

1. **Whole Foods:** The diet promotes the consumption of whole, unprocessed foods. It encourages individuals to choose organic, grass-fed, and wild-caught sources of meat and to opt for fresh, locally sourced fruits and vegetables whenever possible.

2. **Protein Emphasis:** Protein plays a central role in the Paleo Diet, with lean meats, poultry, and fish being the primary sources. These foods are rich in essential amino acids and provide a sense of satiety.

3. **Carbohydrate Sources:** Carbohydrates in the Paleo Diet come primarily from non-starchy vegetables, fruits, and nuts. These foods are low on the glycemic index and provide a steady source of energy.

4. **Elimination of Grains and Legumes:** Grains and legumes are excluded from the diet due to their relatively recent introduction in human history and the presence of anti-nutrients. Advocates argue that eliminating these foods can

reduce inflammation and improve gut health.

5. **Dairy Exclusion:** Dairy products are typically avoided, as they were not part of the Paleolithic diet and can be problematic for individuals with lactose intolerance or sensitivity to dairy proteins.

6. **Emphasis on Healthy Fats:** The diet encourages the consumption of healthy fats, such as those found in avocados, nuts, and fatty fish. These fats provide essential fatty acids and support overall health.

7. **Minimization of Processed Foods:** Processed foods high in refined sugars, artificial additives, and trans fats are

discouraged as they are believed to contribute to various health issues.

8. **Focus on Nutrient Density:** The diet promotes nutrient-dense foods that provide a wide range of essential vitamins, minerals, and other micronutrients.

Paleo Diet is a dietary approach that seeks to align modern eating habits with the presumed dietary patterns of our ancient ancestors. Its principles emphasize the consumption of whole, natural foods while excluding or minimizing processed and modern agricultural products. Advocates of the Paleo Diet believe that by following these principles, individuals can achieve better overall health, maintain a healthy body weight, and reduce the risk of chronic diseases.

# CHAPTER 2

# Foods Allowed on the Paleo Diet

## 2.1 Lean Meats

Lean meats are a cornerstone of the Paleo Diet. This category includes a variety of animal proteins that are low in fat, making them a valuable source of essential nutrients and high-quality protein. Some of the lean meats typically consumed on the Paleo Diet include:

- **Grass-fed and pasture-raised meats:** These are preferred because they tend to have a healthier fatty acid profile and

are free from added hormones
and antibiotics. Common
choices include beef, lamb, and
bison.

- **Poultry:** Chicken and turkey
  are lean sources of protein that
  are compatible with the Paleo
  Diet. It's advisable to opt for
  organic or free-range poultry
  when possible.

- **Game meats:** Wild game, such
  as venison, elk, and boar, are
  considered excellent choices for
  their natural, low-fat content.

- **Lean cuts:** Regardless of the
  type of meat chosen, it's
  recommended to select lean
  cuts to minimize saturated fat
  intake. Examples include
  sirloin, tenderloin, and skinless
  poultry.

Lean meats are a rich source of protein, essential amino acids, vitamins (especially B vitamins), and minerals like iron and zinc. They are essential for muscle health, energy production, and overall well-being within the framework of the Paleo Diet.

## 2.2 Fish and Seafood

Fish and seafood are another vital component of the Paleo Diet. They offer a wealth of essential nutrients and are known for their heart-healthy omega-3 fatty acids. Common fish and seafood options adhering to the Paleo guidelines include:

- **Fatty fish:** Examples include salmon, mackerel, sardines, and trout. These are especially prized for their omega-3 content, which supports brain health and reduces inflammation.

- **White fish:** Varieties like cod, haddock, and flounder are lower in fat but provide an excellent source of protein and essential nutrients.

- **Shellfish:** Shrimp, crab, clams, and mussels are Paleo-friendly choices that offer a good protein source along with essential minerals like zinc and selenium.

Consuming fish and seafood can be beneficial for heart health, brain function, and overall well-being. Their omega-3 fatty acids are recognized for their anti-inflammatory properties.

## 2.3 Fruits

Fruits are a welcome addition to the Paleo Diet due to their natural sweetness and abundance of vitamins, minerals, antioxidants, and dietary fiber. While the diet encourages fruit consumption, it's essential to prioritize fresh, whole fruits and limit the intake of dried fruits or fruit juices, which can be concentrated sources of sugar. Some Paleo-approved fruits include:

- **Berries:** Blueberries, strawberries, raspberries, and blackberries are rich in antioxidants and vitamins while being relatively low in sugar.

- **Citrus fruits:** Oranges, lemons, limes, and grapefruits provide a burst of vitamin C and refreshing flavors.

- **Tropical fruits:** Moderation is key, but fruits like mangoes, pineapples, and papayas can be enjoyed on occasion.

- **Apples and pears:** These fruits are abundant in fiber and a variety of vitamins.

- **Avocado:** While botanically a fruit, avocados are an excellent source of healthy fats and fiber and are often included in the Paleo Diet.

Fruits are not only a delicious source of natural sweetness but also provide essential vitamins, minerals, and antioxidants. They contribute to a well-rounded Paleo diet, helping to meet nutritional needs while satisfying the desire for a sweet treat.

## 2.4 Vegetables

Vegetables are a vital component of the Paleo Diet, providing a rich array of essential nutrients, vitamins, minerals, and dietary fiber. The diet encourages the consumption of a wide variety of fresh, non-starchy vegetables. Here are some examples of vegetables that align with the Paleo Diet:

- **Leafy greens:** Spinach, kale, collard greens, and Swiss chard are excellent sources of vitamins (especially vitamin K), minerals, and antioxidants.

- **Cruciferous vegetables:** Broccoli, cauliflower, Brussels sprouts, and cabbage are known for their cancer-fighting properties and nutritional value.

- **Root vegetables:** While starchy vegetables like potatoes are generally avoided, Paleo-friendly options include carrots, beets, and sweet potatoes, which are rich in vitamins and fiber.

- **Bell peppers:** These are a good source of vitamin C and come in various colors, each offering a slightly different nutrient profile.

- **Zucchini, eggplant, and tomatoes:** These vegetables are versatile and can be used in a wide range of Paleo recipes.

- **Onions and garlic:** These add flavor to dishes while providing health benefits, such as potential immune system support.

Including a variety of colorful vegetables in your diet is essential for getting a broad spectrum of nutrients. They are low in calories and high in dietary fiber, which supports digestive health and helps you feel full and satisfied.

## 2.5 Nuts and Seeds

Nuts and seeds are valued components of the Paleo Diet as they offer a balance of healthy fats, protein, vitamins, and minerals. However, portion control is advisable, as these foods are energy-dense. Some commonly consumed nuts and seeds on the Paleo Diet include:

- **Almonds:** Rich in vitamin E, magnesium, and healthy monounsaturated fats.

- **Walnuts:** Known for their omega-3 fatty acids and antioxidants.

- **Cashews:** A source of copper and magnesium, but they should be enjoyed in moderation due to their higher carbohydrate content.

- **Macadamia nuts:** These are particularly low in omega-6 fatty acids and are a good source of monounsaturated fats.

- **Pecans:** A good source of fiber and various vitamins and minerals.

- **Sunflower seeds:** Rich in vitamin E and other nutrients, they can be used for snacking or as salad toppers.

- **Chia seeds and flaxseeds:**
  These are high in dietary fiber,
  omega-3 fatty acids, and can be
  added to smoothies or used in
  baking.

Nuts and seeds can be incorporated
into the Paleo Diet to add texture,
flavor, and valuable nutrients to meals
and snacks. However, it's important to
consume them in moderation, as they
are calorie-dense and can contribute
to calorie excess if not portioned
carefully.

Incorporating a variety of vegetables,
nuts, and seeds into the Paleo Diet
ensures a diverse and balanced intake
of essential nutrients, helping to
maintain good health and overall
well-being while adhering to the
dietary principles of this approach.

# CHAPTER 3

# Foods to Avoid

## 3.1 Grains and Cereals

One of the central tenets of the Paleo Diet is the exclusion of grains and cereals. The rationale behind this exclusion is based on the idea that grains and cereals, which became a significant part of the human diet with the advent of agriculture, may not be well-suited to the human body due to several reasons:

- **Anti-nutrients:** Grains contain compounds like lectins, phytates, and gluten, which can interfere with nutrient absorption and lead to digestive

discomfort for some
individuals.

- **High glycemic index:** Many grains have a high glycemic index, leading to rapid spikes in blood sugar levels, potentially contributing to insulin resistance and weight gain.

- **Inflammatory potential:** Some grains, particularly those containing gluten, can be inflammatory and may exacerbate conditions like celiac disease or non-celiac gluten sensitivity.

Common grains and cereals to avoid on the Paleo Diet include:

- **Wheat:** This includes all wheat products such as bread, pasta, and most breakfast cereals.

- **Corn:** Corn products, including corn syrup and corn-based snacks.

- **Rice:** Both white and brown rice are excluded from the diet.

- **Oats:** Rolled oats, oatmeal, and oat-based products are not included.

- **Barley, rye, and other gluten-containing grains:** These grains and their byproducts should be avoided.

- **Quinoa and amaranth:** While often considered healthy, they are not part of the Paleo Diet due to their seed-like nature and potential for digestive irritation.

# 3.2 Legumes

Legumes, including beans, lentils, and peanuts, are also excluded from the Paleo Diet. The reasons for avoiding legumes are similar to those for grains and cereals:

- **Anti-nutrients:** Legumes contain compounds like lectins and phytates that can inhibit nutrient absorption and potentially cause digestive issues.

- **Protease inhibitors:** Some legumes contain protease inhibitors that can interfere with protein digestion.

- **Carbohydrate content:** Legumes are relatively high in carbohydrates, which can lead to fluctuations in blood sugar levels.

Common legumes to avoid on the Paleo Diet include:

- **Beans:** This category includes black beans, kidney beans, pinto beans, and other varieties.

- **Lentils:** All types of lentils are excluded.

- **Peas:** Both green and yellow peas are not part of the diet.

- **Peanuts:** Despite the name, peanuts are actually legumes, and they are not considered Paleo-friendly.

- **Soybeans:** This includes soy products like tofu, tempeh, and soybean oil.

## 3.3 Dairy Products

Dairy products are generally avoided on the Paleo Diet. The rationale behind this exclusion is based on the fact that early humans did not practice dairy farming, and the consumption of dairy products only became widespread after the domestication of animals. Additionally, dairy products can be problematic for many individuals due to lactose intolerance or sensitivity to dairy proteins. Key reasons to avoid dairy on the Paleo Diet include:

- **Lactose:** Lactose, the sugar in milk, can be poorly tolerated by many adults, leading to digestive discomfort.

- **Casein and whey:** Some individuals may be sensitive to the proteins found in dairy, such as casein and whey, which can trigger allergies or intolerances.

- **Insulinotropic effects:** Dairy products can stimulate insulin release, potentially leading to blood sugar spikes.

Common dairy products to avoid on the Paleo Diet include:

- **Milk:** Cow's milk and other animal milks like goat and sheep milk are excluded.

- **Cheese:** All forms of cheese, including hard and soft cheeses.

- **Yogurt:** This includes regular and Greek yogurt.

- **Butter:** While butter is a source of healthy fats, it is not included in the Paleo Diet due to its dairy origin.

It's important to note that some variations of the Paleo Diet, such as the Primal Diet, may allow certain forms of dairy like fermented dairy products (e.g., kefir) or ghee (clarified butter). However, in the strictest interpretation of the Paleo Diet, all dairy is avoided.

## 3.4 Processed Foods

The Paleo Diet strongly discourages the consumption of processed foods. The emphasis is on consuming whole, natural foods that are as close to their original state as possible. Processed foods often contain various additives, preservatives, artificial ingredients, and unhealthy fats. Some common processed foods to avoid on the Paleo Diet include:

- **Fast food:** Burgers, fries, and other fast-food items are typically high in unhealthy trans fats, sugars, and sodium.

- **Packaged snacks:** This category includes chips, crackers, cookies, and other snack foods that are often laden with refined grains, unhealthy fats, and added sugars.

- **Processed meats:** Deli meats, sausages, and bacon often contain preservatives, nitrates, and additives that are not in line with the Paleo Diet principles.

- **Frozen meals:** Many frozen meals are heavily processed and contain high levels of sodium, artificial flavors, and preservatives.

- **Canned soups and sauces:** These often contain added sugars, high sodium content, and artificial additives.

- **Sugary beverages:** Sodas, fruit juices, and sweetened drinks are high in added sugars and are typically not allowed on the Paleo Diet.

- **Processed vegetable oils:** Vegetable oils like soybean, corn, and canola oil are high in omega-6 fatty acids and are not considered healthy fats in the Paleo Diet.

The Paleo Diet places a strong emphasis on consuming foods in their whole, natural form to maximize nutrient intake and minimize exposure to additives and unhealthy substances.

# 3.5 Sugars and Sweeteners

The Paleo Diet discourages the consumption of added sugars and artificial sweeteners. The reasons for avoiding sugars and sweeteners are based on their impact on blood sugar levels, inflammation, and overall health. Common sugars and sweeteners to avoid on the Paleo Diet include:

- **Table sugar:** Also known as sucrose, it is a highly refined and processed sweetener that can lead to rapid spikes in blood sugar.

- **High fructose corn syrup (HFCS):** A common sweetener in processed foods and beverages that is associated with various health issues, including obesity and metabolic syndrome.

- **Artificial sweeteners:** These include aspartame, saccharin, and sucralose, and are typically avoided due to concerns about potential health risks.

- **Honey, maple syrup, and agave nectar:** While these are natural sweeteners, they are relatively high in sugars and are used sparingly on the Paleo Diet.

- **Stevia:** Some versions of the Paleo Diet allow for stevia as a natural, calorie-free sweetener.

Avoiding sugars and sweeteners on the Paleo Diet is aimed at promoting stable blood sugar levels, reducing the risk of chronic diseases, and avoiding foods that can contribute to inflammation and energy fluctuations.

The focus of the Paleo Diet is on real, nutrient-dense foods that support overall health, and avoiding processed foods, sugars, and sweeteners aligns with these principles.

# CHAPTER 4

# Benefits of the Paleo Diet

Certainly, here's an overview of the potential benefits of the Paleo Diet, including weight loss, improved blood sugar control, better digestive health, increased nutrient intake, and enhanced energy levels:

## 4.1 Weight Loss

Weight loss is one of the most commonly reported benefits of the Paleo Diet. The diet promotes the consumption of whole, unprocessed foods that are generally lower in calories and refined carbohydrates compared to the typical Western diet. Additionally, the emphasis on protein and healthy fats can increase feelings of fullness and reduce overall calorie intake. This combination of factors may lead to weight loss for individuals following the Paleo Diet.

Moreover, the reduction in processed foods, sugars, and unhealthy fats may help combat overeating and cravings, leading to more sustainable weight management. The Paleo Diet's focus on nutrient-dense foods can support long-term weight control and a healthy body composition.

## 4.2 Improved Blood Sugar Control

The Paleo Diet can contribute to improved blood sugar control, making it a potentially beneficial choice for individuals with diabetes or those at risk of developing the condition. By excluding high-glycemic foods like grains and sugars, the diet helps stabilize blood sugar levels and reduce the risk of insulin resistance. The emphasis on fiber-rich vegetables and low-glycemic fruits further supports steady energy levels and may help prevent blood sugar spikes and crashes.

A consistent, balanced intake of carbohydrates from vegetables, combined with the diet's high-protein content, may help regulate blood glucose and reduce the need for insulin or other diabetes medications for those with diabetes.

## 4.3 Better Digestive Health

Many individuals report improvements in digestive health when following the Paleo Diet. This is due in part to the exclusion of grains and legumes, which contain compounds like lectins and phytates that can interfere with nutrient absorption and cause digestive discomfort for some people. By eliminating these potentially problematic foods, individuals may experience reduced bloating, gas, and gastrointestinal distress.

The focus on fiber-rich vegetables and fruits also supports healthy digestion by promoting regular bowel movements and a balanced gut microbiome. The consumption of fermented foods, such as sauerkraut and kimchi, can further enhance digestive health by providing beneficial probiotics.

## 4.4 Increased Nutrient Intake

The Paleo Diet encourages the consumption of nutrient-dense foods, including lean meats, fish, vegetables, and fruits. These whole foods are rich in essential vitamins, minerals, and antioxidants, which can promote overall health and well-being. By avoiding highly processed and nutrient-poor foods, individuals following the Paleo Diet are more likely to meet their daily nutritional needs.

Lean meats are excellent sources of high-quality protein and important nutrients like iron and zinc.

Vegetables and fruits are packed with vitamins, minerals, and antioxidants that support various bodily functions and help protect against chronic diseases. Nuts and seeds provide healthy fats, fiber, and a range of micronutrients. The Paleo Diet's nutrient-rich profile can contribute to better overall health.

## 4.5 Enhanced Energy Levels

Many individuals who adopt the Paleo Diet report increased energy levels and reduced feelings of fatigue. This could be attributed to several factors:

- Stable blood sugar levels: By avoiding high-glycemic foods and sugar-laden snacks, the Paleo Diet helps maintain steady energy throughout the day, reducing the energy crashes often associated with consuming refined carbohydrates.

- Improved sleep: The diet's emphasis on whole, nutrient-dense foods can positively affect sleep quality, leading to better energy levels during waking hours.

- Reduced inflammation: By eliminating potentially inflammatory foods like grains, legumes, and processed items, the diet may reduce chronic inflammation, which can sap energy.

- Healthy fats: The inclusion of healthy fats from sources like avocados, nuts, and fatty fish can provide a sustained source of energy.

Overall, the Paleo Diet's emphasis on whole, natural foods and the exclusion of potential energy-draining culprits can contribute to enhanced energy levels and improved vitality for many individuals.

It's important to note that the specific benefits of the Paleo Diet can vary from person to person, and individual results may depend on factors such as personal health, adherence to the diet, and lifestyle. Before making any significant dietary changes, it's advisable to consult with a healthcare professional or registered dietitian to ensure that the diet aligns with your health and nutritional goals.

# CHAPTER 5

# Criticisms and Controversies

## 5.1 Lack of Scientific Consensus

One of the primary criticisms of the Paleo Diet is the lack of robust scientific consensus regarding its long-term health effects. While some studies suggest potential benefits, such as weight loss and improved metabolic markers, the evidence is often limited in scope and duration. Critics argue that more rigorous, long-term research is needed to definitively establish the diet's health outcomes, especially in comparison to other dietary approaches.

Additionally, there is debate surrounding the accuracy of the diet's historical premise. Some anthropologists and archaeologists argue that our knowledge of Paleolithic diets is incomplete, making it challenging to accurately replicate the ancestral diet. This lack of historical precision contributes to the skepticism regarding the diet's claims.

## 5.2 Sustainability Concerns

Another criticism of the Paleo Diet pertains to its sustainability and environmental impact. The diet's emphasis on animal protein can raise concerns about overconsumption of meat, which is associated with greenhouse gas emissions, deforestation, and other environmental issues. Critics argue that promoting greater meat consumption can exacerbate these problems and may not be ecologically responsible in a world facing environmental challenges.

In response to these concerns, proponents of the diet have advocated for ethical and sustainable sourcing of animal products, such as grass-fed, pasture-raised, and wild-caught options. However, the broader impact of a meat-centric diet on the environment remains a point of contention.

## 5.3 Nutrient Gaps

Detractors of the Paleo Diet also raise concerns about potential nutrient gaps, particularly regarding calcium and vitamin D. The exclusion of dairy products, a primary source of these nutrients in many diets, can lead to deficiencies if not adequately replaced with alternative sources. Critics argue that maintaining bone health and preventing osteoporosis may be more challenging without dairy consumption.

Additionally, the diet's restriction of grains and legumes, which are sources of dietary fiber and certain vitamins, may require careful planning to ensure an adequate intake of these nutrients.

However, proponents of the Paleo Diet assert that careful food selection can mitigate these concerns, as they advocate for nutrient-rich foods like leafy greens, nuts, seeds, and bone-in fish that can provide calcium, vitamin D, and other essential nutrients.

## 5.4 Adaptability and Practicality

The practicality and adaptability of the Paleo Diet are often criticized. Some individuals find it challenging to adhere to the strict guidelines of the diet, especially in modern, fast-paced lifestyles. Critics argue that the diet can be socially isolating and inconvenient, as it requires avoiding many commonly available and convenient foods.

The cost of purchasing high-quality, organic, and grass-fed meat and other Paleo-compliant foods can be prohibitive for some individuals. This cost factor can make the diet inaccessible to those on a tight budget.

In response to these concerns, proponents of the diet suggest that the core principles of the Paleo Diet can be adapted to individual needs and preferences. They recommend that people make choices that align with their values, health goals, and budget. Additionally, they argue that the long-term health benefits can outweigh the initial challenges of adapting to the diet.

Paleo Diet is not without its share of criticisms and controversies. These range from concerns about scientific validation and sustainability to debates about nutrient adequacy and practicality. While the diet has gained popularity and has numerous adherents, it remains a subject of ongoing discussion and debate in the fields of nutrition and public health. Individuals considering the diet should carefully weigh these criticisms and seek guidance from healthcare professionals or dietitians when making dietary decisions.

# CHAPTER 6

# Getting Started with the Paleo Diet

## 6.1 Planning Your Meals

Starting the Paleo Diet involves careful meal planning to ensure you're getting a balanced and nutritious diet while adhering to the diet's principles. Here are some steps to help you get started:

**Identify Paleo-Friendly Foods:**

- Familiarize yourself with the foods that are allowed on the Paleo Diet, such as lean meats, fish, vegetables, fruits, nuts, and seeds.

- Make a list of your favorite Paleo-compliant foods to incorporate into your meals.

**Create a Meal Plan:**

- Plan your meals for the week. This includes breakfast, lunch, dinner, and snacks.

- Ensure variety by incorporating different proteins, vegetables, and fruits in your plan.

- Think about portion sizes and the balance of macronutrients (protein, fats, and carbohydrates) in each meal.

**Batch Cooking:**

- Consider batch cooking on weekends or when you have

more time. Prepare larger
portions of Paleo-friendly
dishes and store them for easy
access during the week.

- This can save time and ensure
  you always have Paleo options
  readily available.

**Meal Prep:**

- Prepare snacks and meals for
  the week to reduce the
  temptation of reaching for non-
  Paleo options when you're busy
  or on the go.

- Invest in meal prep containers
  to make it convenient to portion
  your meals.

**Seek Inspiration:**

- Look for Paleo recipes in
  cookbooks, online resources,
  and social media. There are

numerous creative and delicious Paleo recipes to keep your meals interesting.

- Plan themed nights (e.g., Mexican, Asian, Mediterranean) to keep your diet exciting.

**Track Your Progress:**

- Consider keeping a food diary to track your meals, how you feel, and any noticeable changes in your health and well-being.

- This can help you identify which foods work best for you and adjust your meal plan accordingly.

- 

# 6.2 Grocery Shopping

Once you've planned your Paleo meals, it's time to hit the grocery store. Here's how to make your shopping experience more efficient and aligned with the Paleo Diet:

**Prepare a Shopping List:**

- Create a detailed shopping list based on your meal plan. This ensures that you purchase the ingredients you need and reduces the chances of buying non-Paleo items on impulse.

- Categorize your list by food groups to make shopping easier.

**Focus on Fresh Produce:**

- Spend a significant portion of your time in the fresh produce section. Choose a variety of colorful vegetables and fruits to get a range of nutrients.

- Opt for organic options when possible, especially for the "Dirty Dozen" items with higher pesticide residues.

**Shop the Perimeter:**

- In many grocery stores, the perimeter is where you'll find fresh, whole foods like meats, seafood, fruits, and vegetables. Stick to the perimeter as much as possible to avoid processed foods in the central aisles.

**Read Labels:**

- When buying packaged foods, carefully read the labels to ensure they meet the Paleo criteria. Look for products with

minimal ingredients and no
added sugars, grains, or dairy.

## Consider Alternative Aisles:

- Explore sections like the nut
  and seed aisle for healthy
  snacks or the gluten-free aisle
  for Paleo-friendly options like
  almond flour and coconut milk.

## Avoid Temptations:

- Stay focused on your shopping
  list and try to avoid aisles with
  non-Paleo items like bread,
  pasta, and processed snacks.

## Bulk Buying:

- Purchase non-perishable items
  like nuts, seeds, and canned
  goods in bulk to save money
  and reduce the frequency of
  shopping trips.

**Stay Hydrated:**

- Don't forget to hydrate while shopping. Carry a water bottle with you to stay refreshed and reduce the temptation to buy sugary beverages.

By planning your meals and being strategic about grocery shopping, you can successfully transition to the Paleo Diet and make it a sustainable part of your lifestyle. Over time, you'll become more familiar with your favorite Paleo foods and develop a routine that suits your individual tastes and needs.

# 6.3 Meal Preparation Tips

Meal preparation is a crucial aspect of successfully following the Paleo Diet.

Here are some tips to help you prepare your meals effectively:

1. **Plan Your Meals:** As mentioned earlier, create a weekly meal plan. This will not only save you time but also help you stick to your dietary goals.

2. **Batch Cooking:** Consider cooking larger batches of proteins like chicken, beef, or salmon, and store them in the refrigerator or freezer. This will make it easy to add protein to your meals throughout the week.

3. **Chop and Wash Veggies in Advance:** Spend some time washing and chopping vegetables in advance. Store them in airtight containers in

the fridge for quick and easy access.

4.  **Prepare Snacks:** Have Paleo-friendly snacks readily available. Nuts, seeds, sliced vegetables, and homemade Paleo energy bars can help you avoid reaching for non-compliant snacks.

5.  **Experiment with Spices:** Spices and herbs can add a lot of flavor to your dishes. Experiment with different combinations to keep your meals interesting.

6.  **Use Healthy Fats:** Cook with healthy fats like coconut oil, olive oil, and avocado oil. These fats are staples of the Paleo Diet and add flavor to your dishes.

7. **Keep Stocked Pantry:**
Maintain a well-stocked pantry
with items like canned tuna,
canned vegetables, and staples
like almond flour, coconut
flour, and coconut milk for
convenient meal preparation.

8. **Pack Meals:** If you're often on
the go, invest in high-quality
containers to pack your Paleo
meals. Having prepared meals
with you will help you resist
the temptation of non-
compliant options.

9. **Stay Hydrated:** Don't forget to
drink plenty of water
throughout the day to stay well-
hydrated.

10. **Listen to Your Body:** Pay
attention to your body's hunger
and fullness cues. The Paleo

Diet encourages intuitive eating, which means eating when you're hungry and stopping when you're satisfied.

## 6.4 Sample Meal Plan

Here's a sample one-day meal plan to give you an idea of what a day on the Paleo Diet might look like:

**Breakfast:**

- Scrambled eggs with spinach, tomatoes, and mushrooms sautéed in olive oil.

- A side of fresh berries (e.g., strawberries and blueberries).

**Lunch:**

- Grilled chicken breast with a mixed salad (lettuce, cucumbers, bell peppers, and onions) drizzled with a balsamic vinaigrette dressing.

- A serving of guacamole with carrot and cucumber sticks for dipping.

**Snack:**

- A small handful of almonds and walnuts.

- Sliced apple with almond butter.

**Dinner:**

- Baked salmon with a lemon and dill sauce.

- Steamed broccoli and cauliflower florets.

- A side of roasted sweet potatoes seasoned with rosemary.

**Snack (if needed):**

- A few cherry tomatoes or baby carrots.

This is just a sample, and you can customize your meals based on your preferences and dietary needs. It's important to prioritize whole, nutrient-dense foods and avoid grains, legumes, dairy, processed foods, and added sugars when planning your meals. Over time, you can experiment with different ingredients and recipes to make the Paleo Diet work for you.

# CHAPTER 7

# Paleo Diet and Exercise

## 7.1 Physical Activity Recommendations

The Paleo Diet is often associated with an active and healthy lifestyle. While the diet itself can provide various health benefits, including improved energy levels and weight management, it is typically paired with a commitment to regular physical activity. Here are some physical activity recommendations:

1. **Mix of Activities:** Aim for a well-rounded mix of activities, including cardiovascular

exercise, strength training, and flexibility exercises. This combination promotes overall fitness and health.

2. **Cardiovascular Exercise:** Engage in regular cardiovascular activities like running, cycling, swimming, or brisk walking. These exercises help improve your heart health, stamina, and can aid in weight management.

3. **Strength Training:** Incorporate strength training into your routine. This can include weightlifting, bodyweight exercises, or resistance band workouts. Building muscle not only boosts metabolism but also supports overall health.

4. **Flexibility and Mobility:**
   Don't neglect flexibility and
   mobility exercises, such as
   yoga or stretching routines.
   These can help improve your
   range of motion, prevent injury,
   and reduce muscle tension.

5. **Consistency:** Consistency is
   key to reaping the benefits of
   exercise. Aim to make physical
   activity a regular part of your
   routine, ideally most days of
   the week.

6. **Listen to Your Body:** Pay
   attention to your body's signals.
   Rest when needed, and don't
   push yourself to the point of
   exhaustion or injury.

7. **Outdoor Activities:** Whenever
   possible, consider outdoor
   activities that align with the

Paleo lifestyle. Activities like hiking, trail running, and outdoor sports can be enjoyable ways to stay active while connecting with nature.

## 7.2 Combining Paleo with Exercise

Here are some tips for effectively combining the Paleo Diet with your exercise routine:

1. **Balanced Nutrition:** Ensure you're consuming a balanced diet that provides the necessary energy and nutrients for your workouts. Incorporate carbohydrates from fruits and vegetables to support your physical activity.

2. **Pre-Workout Meals:** Eat a balanced meal a few hours before your workout. Include a source of protein, healthy fats, and carbohydrates. This provides sustained energy for your exercise session.

3. **Post-Workout Nutrition:** After your workout, have a meal or snack that includes protein to support muscle recovery and carbohydrates to replenish glycogen stores.

4. **Hydration:** Stay well-hydrated before, during, and after your workouts. Water is crucial for optimal exercise performance and recovery.

5. **Supplements:** Some athletes on the Paleo Diet use supplements like protein

powders, creatine, or branched-chain amino acids to support their training. Consult with a healthcare professional or dietitian before using supplements to ensure they align with your dietary and fitness goals.

6. **Timing:** Experiment with the timing of your meals in relation to your workouts. Some people find that eating a balanced meal 2-3 hours before exercise works best, while others prefer a smaller snack closer to their workout time.

7. **Recovery:** Adequate rest and recovery are essential for muscle repair and overall well-being. Ensure you're getting enough sleep, and incorporate

rest days into your exercise
routine to prevent overtraining.

8. **Paleo-Friendly Snacks:** Plan
   for Paleo-friendly post-workout
   snacks, such as a serving of
   mixed nuts or a piece of fruit,
   which can provide the right
   balance of nutrients to support
   recovery.

Remember that the effectiveness of
your diet and exercise plan depends
on individual factors such as your
goals, fitness level, and dietary
preferences. It's important to adapt
your nutrition and exercise to meet
your specific needs and consult with a
healthcare professional or a registered
dietitian to ensure you're following a
well-rounded and balanced approach
to health and fitness.

# 7.3 Fitness Benefits

The Paleo Diet is often associated with several fitness benefits due to its focus on whole, nutrient-dense foods and its avoidance of processed items, grains, and added sugars. While individual results may vary, the following are some of the potential fitness benefits of the Paleo Diet:

1. **Improved Body Composition:** The Paleo Diet emphasizes lean protein sources, which can support muscle growth and maintenance. This can contribute to improved body composition and a higher percentage of lean muscle mass compared to body fat.

2. **Weight Management:** Many people report weight loss or weight maintenance on the

Paleo Diet, attributed to the lower calorie density of whole foods, reduced consumption of processed items, and the natural satiety of high-protein and high-fiber meals.

3. **Steady Energy Levels:** The diet's avoidance of refined carbohydrates and sugars can help stabilize blood sugar levels, leading to sustained energy throughout the day. This can improve your endurance and stamina during workouts.

4. **Enhanced Recovery:** The focus on nutrient-dense foods means you're providing your body with essential vitamins, minerals, and antioxidants, which can support post-workout recovery and reduce muscle soreness.

5. **Heart Health:** The diet's emphasis on healthy fats, lean proteins, and plenty of fruits and vegetables can support cardiovascular health by reducing the risk of heart disease.

6. **Reduced Inflammation:** By eliminating potentially inflammatory foods, such as grains and processed items, the Paleo Diet may help reduce chronic inflammation, which can negatively impact exercise performance and recovery.

7. **Digestive Health:** Many individuals experience improved digestion and reduced bloating or gastrointestinal distress when following the Paleo Diet, which

can enhance comfort during workouts and physical activity.

8. **Mental Clarity:** A diet rich in nutrient-dense foods can contribute to mental clarity, focus, and a sense of well-being. This can be beneficial for maintaining motivation and discipline in your fitness routine.

9. **Balanced Macronutrients:** The Paleo Diet encourages a balanced intake of macronutrients, including protein, healthy fats, and carbohydrates. This balanced approach can support overall energy and workout performance.

10. **Adaptability to Athletic Goals:** The Paleo Diet can be

adapted to suit various athletic goals, whether you're a casual fitness enthusiast, a competitive athlete, or someone interested in muscle gain, fat loss, or endurance sports. You can adjust your nutrient ratios to meet your specific needs.

It's important to note that while many people experience these fitness benefits on the Paleo Diet, individual results may differ. Your age, gender, activity level, and personal dietary preferences all play a role in how the diet may impact your fitness and overall health. Before making any significant dietary changes, especially if you have specific fitness goals, consult with a healthcare professional or a registered dietitian to ensure your nutrition plan aligns with your individual needs and objectives.

# CHAPTER 8

# Paleo Diet for Special Populations

The Paleo Diet can be adapted to suit the needs and preferences of various special populations, including athletes, seniors, and individuals with specific health conditions. Here's an overview of how the Paleo Diet can be applied to these groups:

## 8.1 Paleo for Athletes

Athletes often have unique dietary requirements due to their increased energy expenditure and need for proper recovery. The Paleo Diet can be tailored to support their performance and recovery needs:

- **Higher Carbohydrate Intake:** Athletes may need a slightly higher carbohydrate intake compared to the standard Paleo Diet to fuel their workouts. This can include starchy vegetables like sweet potatoes and more fruit.

- **Protein for Muscle Maintenance:** Adequate protein is crucial for muscle maintenance and repair. Athletes should focus on lean meats, poultry, fish, and consider high-quality protein supplements as needed.

- **Healthy Fats for Energy:** While the Paleo Diet already includes healthy fats, athletes may benefit from added fats like avocados, nuts, and seeds to support their energy needs.

- **Post-Workout Nutrition:** After workouts, it's important to consume a balanced meal or snack with a combination of protein and carbohydrates to aid recovery and glycogen replenishment.

- **Hydration:** Proper hydration is essential for athletes. Staying well-hydrated can help maintain performance and prevent dehydration-related issues.

- **Individualized Approach:** Athletes should work with a sports dietitian to customize their Paleo Diet to meet their specific needs, whether they're involved in strength training, endurance sports, or a combination of both.

## 8.2 Paleo for Seniors

For seniors, the Paleo Diet can be adjusted to meet their nutritional requirements while addressing age-related concerns:

- **Adequate Protein:** Seniors need adequate protein to support muscle mass, which can decline with age. Lean meats, fish, and eggs are good sources.

- **Bone Health:** Ensuring an adequate intake of calcium and vitamin D is crucial for maintaining bone health. While dairy is not part of the Paleo

Diet, there are alternative sources of these nutrients, such as leafy greens, bone-in fish, and sun exposure.

- **Fiber and Digestive Health:** Seniors may require more dietary fiber to support digestive health, especially if they experience constipation or other gastrointestinal issues. A variety of vegetables and fruits can provide fiber.

- **Hydration:** Dehydration is a common concern among seniors. It's essential to drink sufficient water throughout the day.

- **Meal Timing:** Some seniors may find it beneficial to space their meals and snacks more evenly throughout the day to maintain energy levels and support digestion.

- **Individualized Needs:** The nutritional needs of seniors can vary widely, so working with a registered dietitian can help customize the Paleo Diet to meet their specific requirements, especially if they have health conditions or dietary restrictions.

# 8.3 Paleo for Health Conditions

The Paleo Diet can be adapted to address various health conditions and dietary restrictions. Here are some considerations for specific health conditions:

- **Autoimmune Conditions:** The Paleo Diet, with its emphasis on anti-inflammatory foods, may benefit individuals with autoimmune conditions. However, the elimination of nightshades or certain nuts may be necessary for some autoimmune conditions.

- **Gluten Sensitivity or Celiac Disease:** The Paleo Diet is naturally gluten-free, making it suitable for individuals with gluten sensitivity or celiac disease.

- **Diabetes:** The Paleo Diet can be customized to manage blood sugar levels. This may include careful selection of carbohydrates and portion control, along with frequent monitoring of blood glucose.

- **Heart Health:** The diet's focus on lean meats, healthy fats, and vegetables can support heart health. Reducing saturated and trans fats is key for individuals with heart conditions.

- **Digestive Disorders:** Some individuals with digestive disorders, like irritable bowel syndrome (IBS), find relief on the Paleo Diet due to the elimination of grains and processed foods. Careful selection of FODMAPs (fermentable carbohydrates) may be necessary.

- **Kidney Disease:** The diet can be modified to limit protein intake for individuals with advanced kidney disease. Consultation with a healthcare professional is crucial in this case.

- **Weight Management:** The Paleo Diet can be effective for weight management and may be customized to meet weight loss or weight gain goals, depending on individual needs.

In all cases, it's important for individuals with specific health conditions to work closely with healthcare professionals and registered dietitians who can tailor the Paleo Diet to address their unique dietary and medical requirements. The diet's flexibility allows for adaptation to individual health and lifestyle needs.

# 8.4 Evolving Trends in Paleo Nutrition

Evolving trends in Paleo nutrition reflect the ongoing evolution of the Paleo Diet and its adaptation to modern lifestyles, scientific research, and emerging food trends. Here are some notable trends in the world of Paleo nutrition:

**1. Personalized Nutrition:** As with many dietary approaches, personalization is becoming a key trend in Paleo nutrition. Individuals are recognizing that one-size-fits-all approaches may not suit everyone. Customization based on individual needs, preferences, and health goals is gaining traction. This includes variations in macronutrient ratios, food choices, and portion sizes within the framework of the Paleo Diet.

**2. Emphasis on Quality Sourcing:**
The emphasis on high-quality sourcing of foods is a growing trend. This includes prioritizing organic, grass-fed, pasture-raised, and sustainably sourced animal products. The focus is not only on the type of food but also how it was raised or produced.

**3. Inclusion of Fermented Foods:**
Fermented foods, such as sauerkraut, kimchi, and kombucha, are increasingly recognized for their potential health benefits. These foods can support gut health and digestion and are being integrated into the Paleo Diet as part of a broader focus on gut microbiome health.

**4. Integration of Traditional Diets:**
The Paleo Diet is expanding to incorporate elements of traditional diets from various cultures. These

diets often include foods such as bone broth, organ meats, and offal, which are recognized for their nutrient density.

**5. Sustainable and Ethical Choices:** Sustainability is a growing concern for many people, and this extends to their dietary choices. More individuals following the Paleo Diet are making ethical and sustainable choices by supporting local agriculture, choosing wild-caught seafood, and avoiding foods that contribute to environmental issues.

**6. Technological Advancements:** Technology is playing a role in the evolution of Paleo nutrition. Apps and online resources are making it easier for people to find Paleo-compliant foods, access recipes, and track their dietary choices. This makes it more convenient for individuals to follow the diet while staying connected to the broader Paleo community.

**7. Adaptation to Modern Lifestyles:** Recognizing the demands of modern life, there is a trend toward making the Paleo Diet more adaptable to busy schedules. Meal planning, batch cooking, and the creation of Paleo-friendly convenience foods are becoming more common.

**8. Inclusion of Some Non-Paleo Foods:** Some individuals have adapted the Paleo Diet to include certain non-Paleo foods that align with their goals and preferences. This may include the occasional inclusion of dairy products, rice, or legumes in moderation.

**9. Focus on the Mind-Body Connection:** The mind-body connection is receiving more attention in the context of the Paleo Diet. Practices like mindfulness, stress reduction, and improved sleep are recognized as important components of overall health and are being integrated into the broader Paleo lifestyle.

**10. Hybrid Approaches:** Some people are adopting hybrid approaches that combine elements of the Paleo Diet with other dietary philosophies, such as keto or Mediterranean. These hybrid approaches are intended to leverage the strengths of each diet.

It's important to note that while the Paleo Diet has evolved and adapted over time, it remains a topic of ongoing discussion and research in the field of nutrition. As new evidence emerges and our understanding of dietary science advances, the Paleo

Diet and its trends may continue to evolve to better meet the needs and preferences of individuals seeking a healthful and balanced approach to nutrition.